Mother's and My Way of the Cross

A Meditation Memoir for Caregivers

T. Josephine Lawler, OP

ACTA
Assisting Christians To Act
PUBLICATIONS

Mother's and My Way of the Cross
A Meditation Memoir for Caregivers
by T. Josephine Lawler, OP

Edited by Gregory F. Augustine Pierce
Cover design by Tom A. Wright
Cover art "God Heals Broken Hearts" by Julie Lonneman, TheSpiritSource.com
Typesetting by Desktop Edit Shop, Inc.

Published by ACTA Publications
Assisting Christians To Act
4848 N. Clark Street
Chicago, IL 60640
800-397-2282
www.actapublications.com

Library of Congress Catalog number: 2004117008
ISBN: 0-87946-287-6
Printed in the United States of America
Year 10 09 08 07 06 05
Printing 10 9 8 7 6 5 4 3 2 1

Contents

This book is dedicated to St. Catherine of Siena, who gently and courageously cared for patients in medieval Siena's hospital.

It was my privilege to care for my mother in her final years. I also dedicate these reflections to her and to my father, whose goodness and faithfulness have always inspired me.

Introduction

Let us probe together the mystery and privilege of caring.

Mother's and My Way of the Cross is not a theological treatise about the nature of death. It is a short, devotional reflection about caring for someone when he or she is dying. It uses the death of my mom, a person uncelebrated and uncommemorated by the world, to probe the mystery of dying with hope and faith and love. It also explores how I tried to care for my mother in the last phase of her life's journey. From all that seeking and caring, it is my hope that I learned something, even by my mistakes, that may be helpful to you as you care for another.

In 1989, I moved into Mother's home simply because she needed someone with her. I was working for Catholic Charities in Oakland, California, but I had discerned that to follow Jesus at that time in my life was to respond to my mother in her need and to care for her. She was 91 at the time and in the last stage of her life, although she would live for almost six more years.

Only now can I honestly consider my often faulty ministering to her during those six years. What is the meaning of life in that situation—for me, for her, and perhaps for you and your loved one? I need to reflect especially on the last weeks of her life, when she was in the convalescent hospital. No one—nurses, nurse's aides, her doctor, myself—gave her very good care. We simply didn't know how.

I don't mean that we didn't know how to bathe her, help her with meals, dress her, and so forth. (Although we may have faltered here, too.) I mean that we didn't know how to help her to be comfortable emotionally, psychologically, spiritually; we didn't know how to reassure her, to sense her fears and help allay them; we didn't even know how to meet her physical needs in a way that respected what she wanted and that responded to and acknowledged her dignity.

We are an aging society, yet we don't know how to care well for one another when we get old. We don't know how to understand, love, and simply be with a frail, sick, or mentally wounded loved one. Moreover, our poor efforts and the psychological trauma accompanying them drain us physically, psychologically and spiritually. We read in John 10:10, "I came that they may have life, and have it abundantly," but we caregivers often do not know how to choose abundant life for the people for whom we care and for ourselves.

All of these realizations have led me to share my experiences honestly and openly. You are in a very real sense my dialogue partner. I trust that you will not judge me any more than I will judge you. You will understand when I am unclear or defensive or repeat some things. You will know to take what is helpful to you and leave the rest. When I was with Mother, I eagerly read what other caregivers wrote in my hunger to better understand my own situation. I was so afraid, but aching to support, reassure and love my mother. Now I share my deepest thoughts and prayers with you, knowing that they will be reciprocated and that you in turn will help other caregivers when it is time.

I write about Mother's and my journey as a Way of the Cross. I use the Stations as a "hook" on which to hang these meditations, because I have always found them comforting and challenging at the same time. Somehow they speak to the experience of caregiving in a very direct and helpful way.

Let us probe together the mystery and privilege of caring.

T. Josephine Lawler, O.P.
April 30, 2004 Feast of St. Catherine of Siena
—To whom this little book is dedicated.

Prelude

Think of this brief biography as the prelude to the meditations that follow. It will be helpful to realize that the life of this woman, like most of our lives, was one of hopeful optimism as she faced day-in and day-out existence in a busy world. As with most "ordinary" lives, hers had an extraordinary impact on those who loved her. The reader may want to skim the details and move on to the narrative, reflections and prayers that follow. For in the end, this book is not about my mother and me, it is about your loved one and you. I write of mother's and my shared story because it is the only one I know. But the central theme of this meditation memoir is the hope that emerges in the process of giving care to one we love, and that is a universal experience for all caregivers.

My mother, Josephine, began life on April 12, 1898, in Chicago. Her father, whose family was from Alsace-Lorraine, died when she was an infant. Her mother, Jeanette, came to the United States from the Netherlands with her aunts and uncles when she was a child. Jeanette's uncles returned to Holland because, as one of them said, "You need hands like shovels to work in America." But her aunts stayed. Three of the maiden aunts raised Jeanette and later helped raise Mother, while Jeanette ironed dress shirts in a laundry to support what was certainly a "non-conventional" family.

Among our family photo albums are pictures of Mother in her youth with the group of young girls who were her friends. Several of the photos and pasted-in awards attest to her athletic prowess—she won medals in swimming and diving and played on the award-winning women's basketball team, the Eagles, for Sinai Social Center. (The team insisted on playing "men's rules.") She and her friends frequented a place called the Lincoln Center on the north side of Chicago and in the summer, under Center auspices, went to Clear Lake Camp near Janesville, Wisconsin.

She was bilingual, speaking both English and Dutch. When reminiscing about her experiences in school, Mother marveled at the pole in the corner of her first grade classroom. Students climbed up and slid down the pole when so directed by their teacher. The teacher was amazed at Mother's speed and agility in climbing the pole. "She must have thought she had a monkey," Mother would say.

For a short period, Mother boarded at St. Xavier School on 49th and Cottage Grove Avenue. At Easter time, she received a beautifully colored hard-boiled egg from her mother and great aunts. Treasuring it, she hid it safely in a drawer. Many days went by, and a terrible odor permeated the dorm until one of the Mercy Sisters unearthed the egg.

Chicago's Lake Michigan beaches were Mother's childhood playground. On one occasion she skipped school and swam in the lake in her school clothes. On returning home, she hid her wet clothes in the laundry bag, but her mother discovered them and Mother's escapade.

Another time Mother started home from the beach as the sun was setting. She took a shortcut across a railroad yard. Looking up, she saw the light of a train engine approaching her but could not determine on which track the engine was traveling. She says that she ran faster that day than she ever did in her life.

Mother grew into adulthood reluctantly. After graduating from high school, she worked as a secretary at a time when other young women envisioned themselves exclusively as housewife and mother or at least teacher or nurse. It was probably while she worked at Swift and Company in the Chicago Stock Yards that she met Dad, some time before the United States entered World War I.

On October 30, 1919, Mother and Dad were married. Then followed their four children. While I, the oldest, was still a child, Grandma Jeanette contracted uterine cancer. With Dad's support and encouragement, Mother brought Grandma to our home and cared for her until she died.

Mother was always interested in her children, in our friends, and in our progress in school. As soon as the youngest child was old enough to travel, she persuaded Dad to set aside most of his summer vacation for the family to motor to scenic and historical sites in the United States and Canada. The trips were meant to be part of our complete education. We toured the Appalachian Mountains; we marveled at Niagara Falls, Yellowstone, Bryce Canyon, Pike's Peak, Royal Gorge; and we learned history from visits to places such as Washington, D.C., Hollywood, San Francisco, New York and Quebec.

By the time the youngest child was in first grade, Mother drove the family car. She had asked Dad to teach her to drive, but when he did not have time she grew impatient and took the car out on her own. Driving it into the garage for the night was tricky. She knocked into the wall and loosened some of the bricks. Needless to say, Dad soon took Mother on driving lessons, and she became an expert driver.

During most of each summer, we swam in Lake Michigan. The four of us children got into the car with a neighborhood guest (we took turns inviting a friend) and Mother drove us to a Chicago beach. She taught each of us to swim. A few summers she arranged time at Clear Lake for us (the same camp she had attended in her youth). During one of those summers, she volunteered as one of the camp's leaders.

On Saturdays and school holidays each fall, Mother led us on hikes through the Forest Preserves on the outskirts of Chicago. When the winter cold set in, she packed lunches and took us to nature movies in the basement of the Field Museum of Natural History or supervised us as we experienced the exhibits in Hyde Park's Museum of Science and Industry. When we were in our teens, she occasionally escorted us through the Chicago Art Institute on Michigan Avenue.

The day before Christmas was always magical. We decorated the Christmas tree Dad brought home that day, and I was in wonderment at Mother's creations: a cardboard stage with dancers suspended by thread from the stage ceiling, so that they twirled with the slightest breeze; a mirror skating pond surrounded by a miniature village; a Santa Claus ornament for the top of the tree—all covered with cotton and mica that sparkled like snow.

During high school, I undertook daily reading of the Bible, beginning with page one. As time went on, I probed the Bible for answers to questions being raised by Mother with regard to her faith. (She came from a family that did not profess any religious faith.) I remember, in particular, questions regarding evolution in relation to creation and the very existence of God. Many an evening, after the others went to bed, Mother and I discussed these topics.

In the middle of World War II, Swift and Company moved Dad to California to manage their plant in the Vernon section of Los Angeles. Because of the war, limited travel, and scarce housing on the Pacific coast, Mother and my younger sister stayed in Chicago initially, but eventually Dad found an apartment and Mother and my sister joined him.

Mother was lonesome for Chicago and the friends she knew there. She attended art classes and painted many beautiful scenes on canvas using oil, and she hammered and etched copper works. Her beautifully framed art pieces graced the walls of the parlor of her home even when I moved in to care for her. (They now add beauty to my own retirement apartment in Santa Cruz.)

Mother took out a membership in the Jewish Community Center near home and began swimming in the pool. She developed a circle of woman friends there. With a small collapsible two-wheel bike in the trunk of her car, she went to the Marina in Venice and rode with her friends. On warm days they swam and sunned at the Marina. Occasionally they vacationed for three or four days in the middle of the week in a spa or resort in the Palm Springs area.

Some of my memories of Mother are of her middle years, when she reached out to relatives who somehow became estranged from the family members closest to them. Not concerned with why they were estranged, she talked "common sense" with each person. "Life is too short to stay angry," she would tell them. A strong-willed person who would clearly state her own position when she was in a conflict, she nevertheless often capitulated to the other person and readily apologized if she was in the wrong.

Finally Dad retired, and he and Mother toured Europe. Mother wrote the story of their treasured Cook's Tour and placed it with black and white snapshots in a zippered notebook.

As he grew older, Dad developed angina. His condition worsened, and Mother became deeply depressed. Years later she told me that she went to a psychiatrist at the advice of her primary physician (Dad's heart specialist). On November 9, 1971, Dad died. I stayed with Mother for several days after the funeral.

She lived for many years on her own, but on at least two occasions she spoke of my assisting her when she became frail. As we walked along Lake Merritt when she visited me in Oakland in 1987, she asked, "What are you going to do when I am feeble?" Taken aback, I responded, "I don't know; you are not feeble yet." Later, during my annual summer visit to her in Los Angeles, she called out the same question one evening from her bedroom. I answered from my room, "I don't know how, but when you need me I shall respond in some way."

Sincerely and appreciatively she said, "That is very reassuring."

With this clipped conversation, we both went to sleep. As time went on, Mother found it increasingly difficult to be alone, especially at night. When I visited her in August 1989, she said, "I think it's time for you to come and be with me."

Chapter One

Living with Decisions

At the end of October 1989, when my mother was 91, I left my home and work in Oakland and moved into Mother's Los Angeles home to care for her. I found living with her comfortable and pleasant.

From the time I was a child, Mother and I had loved, cared about, and trusted one another. Since I knew she would not take advantage of me, I could respond when she said, "I think it's time," and move in to care for her while working for Catholic Charities in the Archdiocese of Los Angeles. (Eventually I left Catholic Charities and began to do retreat work with the elderly.)

I wonder about those among us caregivers who, for whatever reasons, do not relate well with the person or persons we care for. In such a situation, is it realistic and appropriate that we move in with the person needing care or even that we commit ourselves to full-time caregiving? We must remember that we are responsible for ourselves, for our own lives and development, even while we love and care for others.

I think of two Scripture passages that may guide us here: The first is John 15:13: "No one has greater love than this, to lay down one's life for one's friends." The second is Matthew 22:37-40: "You shall love the Lord your God with all your heart, and with all your soul, and with all your mind. This is the greatest and first commandment. And the second is like it: You shall love your neighbor as yourself. On these two commandments hang all the law and the prophets."

Yes, to give one's life to serve another is the ultimate in following Jesus' way. But to care for another depends as much on loving one's self as on loving the other person. Moreover, we are all limited in some ways. Serving Mother as her primary caregiver was limited by my fears, among other factors. I was afraid of not knowing what to do when she was seriously ill and incapacitated, despite my nurse-aid course and certificate and my years of education and accumulating information on aging and caregiving. I was especially afraid that Mother would die at home and I would not know what to do.

I loved Mother, and I wanted to ease her ending years and even her dying, but the prospect of around-the-clock focus on and absorption in caregiving paralyzed me. Moreover, I was physically less and less able to cope with the amazing strength Mother mustered when she was angry and frustrated (I had never been an athlete). There were other realistic concerns. I found it difficult to access the available help and services, and I was threatened by the consequent invasion of my privacy in our typically open California home.

At the very end, I said no to her coming home from the convalescent hospital. I hope and believe I said no because I recognized wherein I am limited. I did love myself, and I did love Mother.

The First Station: Jesus is condemned

We adore you, O Christ, and we bless you;
Because by your holy cross, you have redeemed the world.

Dear Jesus, as we strive to follow your Way, we too have come to a time when we are confronted with intense suffering. We find it difficult to endure this pain, whether physical or psychological, and we anguish over our failings. Let us follow you now in recalling your passion and death. Teach us to follow you in our own passion and dying.

As we caregivers reflect on the unjust condemnation of Jesus, let us think of false accusations we have made or have had made against us. Perhaps even the person we are caring for now was hurt by us or hurt us. Perhaps it was a simple disagreement, but we never worked through the issue and it grew. Maybe our view of each other and of the issue is now distorted and in a "false accusation" state, but we feel that it is too late to resolve things.

Reflecting on the Way of the Cross for Caregivers:

- Do we sometimes stereotype or judge the person we are helping?
- How do our judgments of our loved one affect the quality of our care as experienced by that person?
- If we strove to develop Jesus' unconditional acceptance, compassion, and love for each person, what effect would our striving have on our relationship with the person we serve, even when the person is angry or abusive to us?
- The one we help is a unique person loved into being by God and formed by God into the unique person we now care for. It is this person for whom Jesus was judged and condemned. It is this person whom Jesus, Son of God, loves now and unconditionally.

At the cross her station keeping,
Stood the mournful mother weeping,
Close to Jesus to the last.

—Stabat Mater

Chapter Two

Being Afraid

Early one Thursday morning I was dressing hurriedly to go to Altadena for a Lenten retreat series, when I heard things falling. I went to Mother's room to find her unable to get out of bed to go into the bathroom. I helped her into the bathroom and then back into bed. She was unable to use her right leg or to hold on to furniture with her right hand. I phoned my retreat partner and asked her to facilitate my part of the retreat. I then phoned Mother's doctor.

As soon as he could get away from the office, he came to see Mother. He explained to her that she probably had suffered a stroke. He recommended that she go to the hospital. Mother said, "If you think so, Doctor." But when he was calling for an ambulance, she cried out, "Not now!" so he desisted. Mother agreed to go "tomorrow." In the meantime, I called my sister. She talked to Mother on the phone to persuade her to go to the hospital. Mother said she would leave the house at 1:00 P.M. The next day, she and I rode in the ambulance to St. Vincent's Hospital. My sister followed in her car. Mother had indeed suffered a stroke.

After a week in St. Vincent's, the doctor moved her to the nearby rehabilitation center, where she underwent tests and therapy. My sister or I visited Mother every day, and I washed her clothes and brought what she needed or requested. Mother's residing in the rehabilitation facility did not relieve my time pressures, but did make it possible for me to continue my retreat ministry.

Mother worked hard to regain her ability to walk and use her right hand so that she could return home. Her friendliness charmed the staff, and eventually she did come home. She was of sound mind and articulate in speech; however, she could not walk without a cane or the support of someone's arm, and she never regained full use of her right hand. She had to give up driving her beloved 1984 Plymouth Reliant.

Hesitantly but willingly, I shouldered the increasingly heavy cross of caregiving. All my reading, studying, and experiences relating to older persons simply confirmed that caring for a frail older person and assuring the older person's quality of life were complex, difficult issues. I felt at sea in uncharted waters. I prayed frequently each day that I might know how to minister to Mother, while accepting freely the help and support of others, especially my sister and Mother's neighbor.

In the meantime, Mother shouldered the cross of the periodic and excruciating pain of sciatica in her left leg. She needed her doctor's ministrations but was reluctant to make an appointment. Finally she acquiesced, and I called the doctor's office. When the time came to dress for the visit, however, she reneged and became very agitated. Once in a while, as she raved, she said the doctor would put her in the hospital and that she did not want to be there when my sister came home from her trip to Europe. After supper that day I spoke to Mother about my loss of time for my retreat work because of the unnecessary delay in her going to the doctor. She apologized and admitted that she was afraid of going into the hospital where she could do nothing but stare at the ceiling.

Gradually I was coming to understand that much of Mother's fussing *was* because she was afraid—afraid of terrible sciatic pain, afraid of being alone because something might happen to her, afraid something could happen to me or my sister and we would not be there for her. Perhaps underlying all, she was afraid of the act of dying (not of death itself). She had directed us several times that when she was dying she did not want to receive medications or procedures that would prolong her life, and she had verified her decision in the

"Durable Power of Attorney" that she had signed.

Dying is that strange, awesome, lonely phenomenon that none of us has experienced before it occurs; and Mother could not feel the comfort and reassurance that a person with faith in God might feel. She had converted shortly after marrying my father, but later she began to question. I prayed that, despite my own fears, I might have courage and be able to help and reassure her. Perhaps I might alleviate some of her fear.

The Second Station: Jesus takes up his cross

We adore you, O Christ, and we bless you;
Because by your holy cross, you have redeemed the world.

> *Dear Jesus, as we strive to follow your Way, we too have come to a time when we are confronted with intense suffering. We find it difficult to endure this pain, whether physical or psychological, and we anguish over our failings. Let us follow you now in recalling your passion and death. Teach us to follow you in our own passion and dying.*

As we caretakers think of Jesus during the Agony in the Garden, we cannot help but recognize our agony as well. Jesus pleaded that his Father take away the cup of his Passion and Crucifixion, and we sometimes do the same. But when the cross was imposed on him to carry, he accepted it, and so must we. We may dread the cross of caring for our loved one. We are afraid of the burden, the difficulties, the pain it causes. We don't know how to bear the weight.

Reflecting on the Way of the Cross for Caregivers:
- When we accepted the ministry of caring for our loved one, we accepted and shouldered a cross whose weight we did not know.
- There are unforeseen sufferings that weigh down the cross and rub our shoulders raw—even while there are treasured, joyful moments.

- How do we bear the weight of unforeseen suffering?
- Our constant prayer is that we not shrug off our cross onto others, especially onto the person whom we serve.

Through her heart his sorrow sharing,
All his bitter anguish bearing,
Now at length the sword has passed.
—Stabat Mater

Chapter Three

Making Mistakes

As I wrote about Mother's stroke, I realized that at the time I did not rush her to the nearest hospital emergency room as directed by gerontologists, medical professionals, and everything I have ever read and heard about helping a person who suffered a stroke. Now I ask, Why not?

I delayed partly because I tend to go into denial in dangerous or threatening situations, partly because I react slowly, partly because (by habit) I obeyed Mother and always waited for her to direct me, and partly because I believed that Mother should decide what should be done in her life.

I still feel comfortable with the process by which Mother, my sister, Mother's doctor and I decided to bring Mother to St. Vincent's Hospital. Although she fussed when I was packing her things and resisted when the ambulance was on its way to the house, basically we honored her decisions. That Mother's doctor also honored her wishes, even to setting the time she should leave the house, confirmed my instincts.

It behooves caregivers to communicate, if at all possible, with the person receiving care; even if conferring with the person results in more difficult, less clear decisions. We cannot ignore someone who deserves respect and dignity at all times, and especially at these times.

Even in the midst of emergency situations, I found periods of time when I had to wait for someone or something—the doctor, the ambulance, a return phone call. In my impatience because of the emergency or simply because I could not "waste time," I would fret and worry. Eventually, however, I realized that these were the precious moments I longed for and needed. Perhaps I could take advantage of them, despite the present urgency. I could pray, asking God for help to respond to Mother after the immediate emergency was resolved. I could develop different scenarios that correspond with likely future emergencies, imagining ways to talk over possible situations with Mother in the future.

I suggest that you find time to reflect, pray, and think about your loved one. Be attentive to what he or she communicates both when asked and in casual conversations. Ask for clarification if you are not sure what he or she is telling you.

Gather information on caregiving and on likely emergency situations. Your loved one's primary physician may be a valuable source of information, and you need to know how available he or she is outside of office hours. Phone directories, newspapers, senior centers, and social service agencies offer valuable information. AARP, Area Agency on Aging, Catholic Charities or Catholic Social Service, churches, synagogues, or other faith-based groups can help. People who have had experience with caregiving may offer excellent practical advice. Listen, read, and take notes. File the information you gather where you can find it quickly.

The Third Station: Jesus falls the first time

We adore you, O Christ, and we bless you;
Because by your holy cross, you have redeemed the world.

> *Dear Jesus, as we strive to follow your Way, we too have come to a time when we are confronted with intense suffering. We find it difficult to endure this pain, whether physical or psychological, and we anguish over our failings. Let us follow you now in recalling your passion and death. Teach us to follow you in our own passion and dying.*

As we caregivers imagine the weight of two pieces of wood large enough and strong enough to bear an adult man, we think of how heavy the burden of caregiving can sometimes feel. Just as Jesus, who is model and teacher for his followers, grew weak and fell under the weight of the cross, we feel that sometimes we too may fall. We thank Jesus for accepting his vulnerability and weakness, because that helps us accept ours.

Reflecting on the Way of the Cross for Caregivers:

- We are sorry for our willful misdeeds as a caregiver, but we are just as sorry for our vulnerability and weakness that causes us to fail in our responsibilities and causes pain and sorrow for our loved one.
- We must accept ourselves and our imperfections and failings as caregivers.
- Accepting our failings, how might we minimize practically the ways we harm the person for whom we care?

O how sad and sore distressed,
Was that Mother highly blessed
Of the sole begotten Son.

—Stabat Mater

Chapter 4

Feeling Sorry

I had spoken to Mother about the work time I lost when she balked at going to the doctor and delayed getting herself ready. At other times, I was the one who delayed assisting Mother when she needed it, explaining that I had to do something else at the time.

I thought of my delaying when I reflected on John 2:1-12, which tells about Jesus and Mary at the wedding feast at Cana:

> Dear Jesus, I notice that Mary—like most mothers—expected you, her adult Son, to respond when she pointed out that the wedding couple had run out of wine. You spoke as an adult child often speaks, "Why turn to me? My hour has not come yet." How often do I respond to Mother, "Not now," or "Later," or "I need to do this first." As in your case, my response may be legitimate, but can I help only when I think it is time or when I have planned to respond? True love may be responding on the other person's terms.
>
> Teach me, dear Jesus, how to balance my need for using time as I see best with Mother's need for help "now." You did respond to Mary's plea. Perhaps I should plan to help on Mother's terms when I can do so physically, psychologically and practically. Help me always to respond immediately when she is in an emergency situation, even if her emergencies are frequent or appear to me to be overblown.

When I was scheduled to give a weekend retreat, my sister invited Mother to stay with her, an invitation she often extended to Mother. Mother was reluctant, but I persuaded her to try staying in my sister's home and see whether that arrangement would solve the problem of care for her while I was away. She stayed Friday night. When I phoned again Saturday evening, my sister told me Mother had returned home and that *"it was all right!"*

That Mother returned home that night may have been all right, but we still needed to address the problem of caring for her when I was away. I reflected on Mark 10:21. When a young man asked Jesus, "What must I do to inherit eternal life?" Jesus, looking at him, loved him and said, "Go sell what you own, and give the money to the poor, and you will have treasure in heaven; then come follow me."

Station IV: Jesus and his mother meet

We adore you, O Christ, and we bless you;
Because by your holy cross, you have redeemed the world.

> *Dear Jesus, as we strive to follow your Way, we too have come to a time when we are confronted with intense suffering. We find it difficult to endure this pain, whether physical or psychological, and we anguish over our failings. Let us follow you now in recalling your passion and death. Teach us to follow you in our own passion and dying.*

As we caregivers reflect on Jesus meeting his mother on the way to his death, we reflect on how our loved ones look at us. Just as Jesus must have felt sorry for his mother, how hard it must be for our loved ones to feel that they are the cause of our own work and concern. How often they must feel guilty for demanding our help, even though they need it through no fault of their own. Let us remember that Jesus never wanted to cause his mother pain or sorrow.

Reflecting on the Way of the Cross for Caregivers:

- Are we scared regarding the future because we don't know how to plan?
- Does our loved one resist any kind of help from anyone else but us?
- Are we afraid to make decisions for our loved one because we want the decisions on care to be theirs, but then we are afraid to accept the consequences of their decisions? If left on our own, perhaps we'd risk doing what they want, especially when we have to be away from them. But there are other people's opinions and feelings to be considered.
- What do our loved ones feel when they see how hard we work or have to adjust to our times away from them?

Christ above in torment hangs,
She beneath beholds the pangs
Of her dying glorious Son.

—Stabat Mater

Chapter Five

Getting Away

While returning home on Amtrak from San Diego after meeting with my community of Sisters, I prayed, focusing on my "alone times" in a typical day at home. There was the morning period before Mother arose, the time during her afternoon nap and sometimes during an hour nap in the evening, and the time after she went to bed. When I added up these times, to my surprise, the sum was about four hours a day.

I needed to change my thinking about my time and the interruptions caused by caring for Mother. I needed to consciously recognize and relish my alone times and to value the time I was with Mother. I knew she had so little time left in her life, and I did not want to regret anything after she died.

Still, I needed some respite away from caregiving. Making time to be with my Sisters (who did not reside in the Los Angeles area) was my responsibility as a member of my community, but it also provided needed time away. I loved the times when I was with my congregation. Likewise, planning and preparing for the few retreats I was still able to give offset the stress of giving Mother care while I worked at home. It also left me with some ministry outside the home and assured me that there would be "something there" for me after Mother died and no longer needed me to care for her.

But changing my thinking was not enough. There were still questions: Should Mother ever be alone? What should Mother, my sister, and I do when I was working? I decided to talk again to my sister, to Mother's doctor, and to Mother. I might even ask her to decide among options for care when I was away.

Station V: Simon helps Jesus carry his cross

We adore you, O Christ, and we bless you;
Because by your holy cross, you have redeemed the world.

> *Dear Jesus, as we strive to follow your Way, we too have come to a time when we are confronted with intense suffering. We find it difficult to endure this pain, whether physical or psychological, and we anguish over our failings. Let us follow you now in recalling your passion and death. Teach us to follow you in our own passion and dying.*

This should be called the "Caregiver's Station." Simon was seized and forced to carry Jesus' cross. He had no opportunity to accept or reject helping Jesus, whom he may not even have known. Jesus, in his weakness, would have been grateful for Simon's help, even if he could not articulate his thanks. My Jesus, thank you for accepting the need for help and support from Simon. Help us acknowledge our own weakness and seek help from others when we need it.

Reflecting on the Way of the Cross for Caregivers:

- My generation did not include care for the elderly in their "vocation" plans. Some of us caregivers were psychologically unprepared when the need arose for us to shoulder the cross of caregiving, even if, as was my case, we had studied about older adults and worked professionally with them.
- Are we preparing for the time when we ourselves will need caregivers? How will we find those people? How will we treat them?
- How are we helping future generations to address the needs of the generation ahead of them compassionately?

Is there one who would not weep,
Whelmed in miseries so deep,
Christ's dear mother to behold?

—Stabat Mater

Chapter 6

Being Present

Before supper one evening, Mother told me, "Your sister thinks I should go into a retirement home." Mother was hurt. With my arm around her waist, I responded calmly that she needed someone with her whenever I was away, and we needed to plan for the future.

Mother said she wanted to continue to live with me. She wondered if there was enough money for someone to come into the house to help, especially when I was away. I suggested that we use her monthly Social Security and pension money and not touch her savings. Still she did not agree to my asking someone to come in. We sat on the edge of her bed for a long time talking.

Mother ate little supper that night. After supper she napped. Later, when she prepared for bed, she was very agitated. At 2:45 A.M. I heard her go into the bathroom, and then I heard a loud thud. She had fallen into the tub, pulling the shower curtain with her. I helped her out of the tub. She was not hurt. I felt as sad and helpless as I'm sure she did.

The next night, about every two hours, Mother awakened and called me: "Isn't it time for you to get up and get ready to go to your retreat?" Each time she thought it was midmorning. In her confusion, she finally stumbled around the house, turned up the furnace, and lit the gas stove to make herself tea.

I was appalled and terribly afraid. Having tried to help her and reassure her, I returned to bed following her last agitated wandering, cowered under the covers in fright, and prayed again to know what to do and where to get help in the middle of the night. Some time later, Mother fell asleep and so did I.

I rose early the following morning, dressed for the pre-Lenten retreat I was to give, and then awakened Mother. She was fine and did not remember anything of her pre-dawn activities. However, I phoned my retreat partner and arranged to return home after I facilitated the beginning session of the retreat.

Station VI: Veronica wipes the face of Jesus

We adore you, O Christ, and we bless you;
Because by your holy cross, you have redeemed the world.

> *Dear Jesus, as we strive to follow your Way, we too have come to a time when we are confronted with intense suffering. We find it difficult to endure this pain, whether physical or psychological, and we anguish over our failings. Let us follow you now in recalling your passion and death. Teach us to follow you in our own passion and dying.*

We stand near a woman who watches the pitiful procession to Calvary. Notice her compassion and thoughtfulness. She is a natural caregiver. When she perceives the sweat and blood dripping down Jesus' face, she moves immediately to wipe them away. Jesus, help us not to hesitate to offer what succor we can to our loved one for whom we care—no matter how insignificant the action may seem. We are sorry for the times we turn away and pretend we don't see or hear our loved one's need.

Reflecting on the Way of the Cross for Caregivers:

- How insightful of the authors of the Way of the Cross to memorialize the simple, thoughtful act of a woman we call Veronica.

- Sometimes it is the simplest acts of caregiving that are the most appreciated.
- There is usually not so much a "right" way of caregiving as there is the "loving" way.
- Sometimes being present is the only present that we can give.

Can the human heart refrain
From partaking in her pain
In that mother's pain untold?
—Stabat Mater

Chapter 7

Accepting Limitations

In the next two months, aware that she easily became confused, Mother worked hard at orienting herself. One afternoon, when she awakened from her nap, she was disoriented. After reorienting herself, she worried about her confusion and became uncharacteristically docile. In the evening she asked me many questions as she tried to understand why she had been confused. Feeling compassionate and striving myself to understand, I sat with her, listened, and patiently responded to her.

The feast of indomitable Catherine of Siena arrived in my heart. (I mention Catherine because I admire the compassion with which she cleansed and bound the sores of the sick in Siena's medieval hospital.) I read the gospel for the day, John 6:16-21. In the midst of the stormy sea, Jesus walked on the water to the disciples. They were terrified; but Jesus said, "It is I; do not be afraid." Situations with Mother did frighten me—especially periods when she became disoriented. But what worried me more was my own immobilization when I was afraid yet needed to make decisions on her behalf.

During this period, my superior called to inform me that an apartment was available in Dominican Oaks, the Santa Cruz retirement facility in which a number of our Sisters lived. Mother and I could move there, and I would have the support of a number of Sisters in caring for her.

Even though I was sure Mother would not want to leave her home, I presented the suggestion to her. As I expected, she did not want to move, because she was accustomed to her neighborhood and would find it difficult to adjust to new surroundings and people. She did express concern for me, however, and if I wanted to move to Santa Cruz, she would manage.

That afternoon I heard Mother rise from her nap, but she did not come to my door as usual. I went out and found her sitting quietly in the parlor. I sat down with her and told her that I was not bored living with her, that I did not want to move away from her, and that the work I was doing on retreats was enough for me. Mother said she realized and appreciated how much my sister and I were doing for her, and she thanked me. I have always treasured that conversation. As I realized how frail Mother was, I also recognized how psychologically frail I was.

Station VII: Jesus falls the second time

We adore you, O Christ, and we bless you;
Because by your holy cross, you have redeemed the world.

> *Dear Jesus, as we strive to follow your Way, we too have come to a time when we are confronted with intense suffering. We find it difficult to endure this pain, whether physical or psychological, and we anguish over our failings. Let us follow you now in recalling your passion and death. Teach us to follow you in our own passion and dying.*

How hard it must have been for Jesus to continue bearing the weight of his cross. We feel that sometimes caregiving is so difficult that we fall ourselves. As we provide care to our loved one, we sometimes refuse to accept our limitations. When suffering and stress fell us, we sometimes feel as though the terrible weight of caregiving will never end.

Reflecting on the Way of the Cross for Caregivers:

- How beleaguered both the caregiver and the recipient of care can feel! Often all we have is one another.
- When we need to take care of ourselves, we have to take care of ourselves.
- We are neither God nor superman. We're not even much of a saint most of the time, and our loved one knows this better than anyone else.
- Who will help us realize the sacredness of our relationship with our loved one?

Bruised, derided, cursed, defiled,
She beheld her tender child,
All with bloody scourges rent.

—Stabat Mater

Chapter 8

Deciding to Decide

When I prayed and reflected on Mother's and my way of the cross, I sometimes reached decisions regarding actions I should take. But then I did not follow through, at least not immediately. I remained conscious of those decisions and usually felt guilty because I did not act on my resolve. In some cases, however, when an appropriate situation arose I spontaneously carried out the decision.

Mother was becoming more frail. I treasure many of our conversations, but now, as I remember those conversations, I wish I had encouraged Mother to tell more about her mother and maiden great aunts and about her exploits with her friends. I would like to know more about Dad as she knew him. Not only would I have additional memories to mull over, but Mother may have felt more appreciated and I may have understood her and her reactions to certain situations better.

A cold and cough Mother contracted did not abate, and she did not want to go to the doctor. One night, as we were eating our usual before-bed dessert, she fell asleep in her chair before she had finished her piece of strawberry pie. After I was ready to go to bed, I roused her so that she could rest in bed and not be disoriented when she awakened. But she could not walk. I propped her in the chair and slid it to her bed. Mother said she did not know what was wrong; she said she felt as though she were drugged. Again the next morning, when she wanted to get up, she could not.

The next day was terrible. I acted according to the advice of the gerontological and geriatric professionals. I talked to Mother in the morning and explained that she may have suffered a stroke and perhaps she should go into the nearest emergency room. I talked to my sister, and she started on her way to be with us. The nearest hospital to home was closer to both of us than St. Vincent's, where Mother usually went, so we agreed that I should try to get the HMO, which used both hospitals, to agree to let us take Mother to the closer one. When I called Mother's doctor, I learned that he was on a brief vacation. The replacement doctor would check with the nearest hospital while I called the ambulance. The hospital agreed to accept Mother and then seek approval of the HMO.

The events following the phone calls were nightmarish. First, the ambulance went to the same address on the street one block west of us. Once phone conversations untangled the mistake and the ambulance arrived, I rode with Mother in the ambulance the short three miles, while my sister followed in her car.

The emergency room was crowded. Mother was given a hospital gown and placed on a gurney in a small room. The room was cold, so we asked for blankets. Then we waited and waited. At long intervals someone would enter and do one small bit of preliminary work, as Mother grew more and more agitated. She began to scream and begged, then ordered, us to take her home.

At last she was wheeled to the emergency room doctor. After a while the doctor came back to my sister and me and said Mother had not suffered a stroke but had pneumonia. Mother returned to the room, and we waited. It was long past her lunchtime, so we asked for lunch for Mother. She ate and drank the sandwich and milk that were brought to the room. We waited. Evening was approaching. Since my sister did not drive after dark, I suggested that she return to her home. Mother and I waited some more.

Suppertime came. I asked about some food for Mother. She would receive a meal when she was admitted to her room, I was told, and she would be assigned to a room as soon as a vacated one was readied.

Finally an aide wheeled her to a room. I asked the nurse for dinner for Mother and was told that she would receive something to eat after the doctor saw her. We waited. Finally the doctor arrived and gently checked Mother. He would see that she received supper. The doctor drove me home.

The next day, about 6:00 A.M., a nurse phoned from the hospital: Mother was very agitated and the nurses could not calm her. Now it was my turn to be agitated: Were not hospital personnel better trained and equipped to work with agitated patients than I was? All I said was that I would be visiting Mother as soon as I could.

A short time later, the doctor called and said the HMO was transferring Mother to St. Vincent's Hospital. My sister and I went to St. Vincent's to find Mother comfortably settled. Frankly, I was relieved that Mother was among people who understood her and knew how to respond.

Station VIII: The women weep for Jesus

We adore you, O Christ, and we bless you;
Because by your holy cross, you have redeemed the world.

> *Dear Jesus, as we strive to follow your Way, we too have come to a time when we are confronted with intense suffering. We find it difficult to endure this pain, whether physical or psychological, and we anguish over our failings. Let us follow you now in recalling your passion and death. Teach us to follow you in our own passion and dying.*

Like these women who followed Jesus faithfully and supported and served him, many caregivers are women. Let us stand with them. We caregivers often must look beyond the present situation, even as we empathize and are present with one who suffers. We must somehow muster energy to look ahead to the time after our caregiving is done.

Reflecting on the Way of the Cross for Caregivers:

- How do we determine the best course of action for our loved one?
- If we do not act immediately, we must determine why we hesitate. Then we need to deliberately place the issue on our "to do later" list, even if we suspect that we are afraid.
- Perhaps you sense that the present is not the time to respond, or you are not ready, or your loved one needs to discuss the issue and be the primary decision-maker.
- Always, always, include the one you care for in decisions that are needed.

For the sins of his own nation
Saw him hang in desolation
Til his spirit forth he sent.

—Stabat Mater

Chapter 9

Letting Go

Mother stayed in St. Vincent's Hospital a week and was very agitated. My sister and I visited several long-term care facilities, and Mother agreed to move into one of them if we found it acceptable and there was enough money.

The day after our conversation about moving to a board and care facility, however, Mother did not know where she was when I visited her. As I was leaving, she asked whether she should come home with me. In all other respects she was perfectly rational. She had even read the Sunday comics and her Agatha Christie mystery novel.

Her mental condition deteriorated rapidly after she was moved to the rehabilitation center for therapy. She was becoming more and more agitated and was disoriented for longer periods of time. My sister and I researched other nursing homes and reserved a bed in the new wing of the St. John of God facility.

Mother wanted to come home and even promised to let her friend next door stay with her when I needed to be away. When I did not agree to bring her home, she felt betrayed: It was her house, and she had a right to live there. I felt terrible. I was not able to help her when she most needed help. I prayed, "Dear Jesus, I grieve for Mother because she is so miserable and mainly because, when rational, she feels as though I let her down. She has been so agitated. Medication is calming her, but her mind is almost gone. Perhaps her situation is too much for her to cope with. Please be with her."

The rehabilitation center staff also floundered; as a result, Mother did not receive the care she needed and was miserable. The very fact that she could not return home seemed to trigger her agitation and disorientation. I prayed that she be reconciled to being cared for away from home. I prayed, too, that I would allow the Spirit to work in Mother and in me, wherever it might lead us.

Station IX: Jesus falls the third time

We adore you, O Christ, and we bless you;
Because by your holy cross, you have redeemed the world.

> *Dear Jesus, as we strive to follow your Way, we too have come to a time when we are confronted with intense suffering. We find it difficult to endure this pain, whether physical or psychological, and we anguish over our failings. Let us follow you now in recalling your passion and death. Teach us to follow you in our own passion and dying.*

When Jesus stumbles and falls a third time, his strength is obviously spent. Yet he wills to rise and force himself to shoulder the cross one more time. How often do we caregivers feel like that? We think that we cannot possibly keep going, and then we do. There is something to be said for just remaining faithful to our commitment, even when we don't have the slightest idea what is the right thing to do.

Reflecting on the Way of the Cross for Caregivers:

- How do we continue to care for our loved one when the person we serve is so weak and helpless that he or she cannot even try?
- Sometimes we ourselves get sick or tired or depressed. Some of us are even getting elderly ourselves.
- How do we replenish our inner resources and the will to continue our loving care?
- Only in the fallen Jesus can we find strength, hope and guidance.

O thou Mother! Font of love,
Touch my spirit from above,
Make my heart with thine accord.
—Stabat Mater

Chapter 10

Being at Peace

I had often thought that John 21:15-19 is relevant to the situation of frail older adults. Now it seemed to relate in a special way to Mother's predicament. The Risen Jesus had cooked breakfast for the disciples on the seashore. Three times Jesus asked Peter if he loved him, and three times Peter had said he did. Jesus asked Peter to care for his lambs and sheep and then continued: "I tell you, when you were younger, you used to fasten your own belt and to go wherever you wished. But when you grow old, you will stretch out your hands, and someone else will fasten a belt around you and take you where you do not wish to go."

I visited Mother one afternoon. She was sleeping in bed with restraints holding her in. After a time, she moaned. Every so often she moaned again. She tried to sit up, so I cranked up the head of the bed. I said several times, "Mother, what's wrong?" She did not rally. When I was leaving, I kissed her forehead and said, "I love you."

The next day she was sitting in her wheel chair in her new dress. At 6:00 P.M. she was fed supper and ate about a third of it. After supper she was helped into bed. At 7:50 P.M., when the nurse checked, she was not breathing and had no pulse.

I thanked the Lord that she was at peace at last. She was 97 years old. Still, I was sad that I was not with her during her last moments and that she was alone when she died. Why had I not recognized that she was dying and stayed later with her on Friday? Why did I remain home on Saturday to wash sheets and towels and clean the house instead of visiting and at least sitting with her? I did not know the answer to these questions.

Station X: Jesus is stripped of his garments

We adore you, O Christ, and we bless you;
Because by your holy cross, you have redeemed the world.

> *Dear Jesus, as we strive to follow your Way, we too have come to a time when we are confronted with intense suffering. We find it difficult to endure this pain, whether physical or psychological, and we anguish over our failings. Let us follow you now in recalling your passion and death. Teach us to follow you in our own passion and dying.*

A soldier pulls off Jesus' clothing. The indignity embarrasses us, and we almost turn our eyes away. How often have our loved ones been stripped of their dignity, and we were powerless to do anything about it? Maybe our own dignity has been compromised by some of the things we have had to do for our loved ones. Dear Jesus, you were robbed of your dignity for all of us. We are sorry for our concern with presenting a good appearance before others instead of worrying about the needs of our loved one. Help us to accept the unmasking of self that our own older years will thrust upon us.

Reflecting on the Way of the Cross for Caregivers:

- Not only is the dying person stripped of all, but those who love the person, especially those who cared most for him or her, also feel stripped and emptied.
- How do we meet the eyes of others who know how difficult our work of caregiving is for us?
- One of the many benefits of caregiving is the honesty it forces upon us.
- Let us give ourselves time to grieve.

Make me feel as thou hast felt;
Make my soul to glow and melt
With the love of Christ my Lord.

—Stabat Mater

Chapter 11

Grieving Our Loss

Although part of me was at peace with Mother's death, I also grieved because I let her down at her hour of most critical need. I prayed:

Mother, I am so sorry I was not with you at the end. I wanted so to alleviate your fright and physical discomfort. You yearned to come home; in fact, you fought to come home. I let you down. I'm terribly sorry! But you know, Mother, that I am weak and that I, too, was terribly afraid. You knew that when you lashed out at me and called me a coward. I really wanted to bring you home and keep you here, protect you, love you.

But I had to be realistic. You never wanted me to be away and you panicked even when I left the house for a few minutes. When others in the hospital cared for you, you called for me so loudly and so often that I knew that part-time in-home help would not really relieve me and make caring for you at home possible.

The mother who ranted and raved was a stranger to me, but I never stopped loving you, for you could not help yourself. I accept you for who you are, and I accept myself for who I am. I just want you to know I loved you then, and I love you now.

Station XI: Jesus is nailed to the cross

We adore you, O Christ, and we bless you;
Because by your holy cross, you have redeemed the world.

> *Dear Jesus, as we strive to follow your Way, we too have come to a time when we are confronted with intense suffering. We find it difficult to endure this pain, whether physical or psychological, and we anguish over our failings. Let us follow you now in recalling your passion and death. Teach us to follow you in our own passion and dying.*

The thing about nails is that they hold things together. Caregiving does too. Despite the pain that we go through with our loved ones, we are tied to them in a way that we are to no others. Their suffering is our suffering, and if they should die a large piece of us dies as well. As Jesus is nailed to his cross, let us be thankful for the nails of love that bind us to our loved ones.

Reflecting on the Way of the Cross for Caregivers:

- What can we do to better minister to the person for whom we care?
- Might we not bear our own pain better by witnessing to the suffering of our loved one?
- Perhaps our patience, and a few gentle reminders, may strengthen our loved one to rely on the God who suffered.
- Death, be not proud. We have overcome you with our love and faith and hope.

Holy Mother pierce me through,
In my heart each wound renew
Of my Savior crucified.

—Stabat Mater

Chapter 12

Saying Goodbye

As my sister and I prepared for Mother's funeral, I prayed that we might celebrate her long life with us. Her Memorial Mass was simple and beautiful.

I continued to live in Mother and Dad's home. Slowly I set neglected areas of the house aright and brought Mother's possessions and personal business to closure. When reading God's admonition to Moses, "The place on which you are standing is holy ground" (Exodus 3:5), I reflected, "I thank you, God, for this place on which I stand. It is holy because it was made holy by the lives of my parents. It is the place you want me to be."

Now as I work, I continually pray and reflect on how we caregivers might help fill the last days of our loved ones with peace and spiritual enrichment. I hear Jesus saying, "Look around you and see how the fields are ripe for harvesting" (John 4:35), and I pray: "Dear Jesus, I see vast fields of older persons ready for their final stage of growth, but there are few who heed or tend to their spiritual needs. Thank you for the opportunity to be of some help. The seed was sown, and it has flowered through your guidance and the self-help of older persons themselves. Please turn the attention of reapers to the abundant harvest standing in readiness."

All of us as human beings are approaching the ultimate goal of our lives, which is eternal life with our God. But the sick and elderly among us are among the most marginalized people in today's fragmented world. It is good that we caregivers are aligning ourselves with them. Even as I was anxious and afraid while caring for Mother, I felt privileged that I could be with her at the end of her life to serve her when she could not help herself, when she was bereft of everything—even the logic of her clear intelligent mind and the strength to care for her own personal needs. I felt privileged that I might serve her, even while I realized that her strong free will had to yield to my judgments and decisions, to the doctor's recommendations, to the ministrations of nurse's aides.

Station XII: Jesus dies on the cross

We adore you, O Christ, and we bless you;
Because by your holy cross, you have redeemed the world.

> *Dear Jesus, as we strive to follow your Way, we too have come to a time when we are confronted with intense suffering. We find it difficult to endure this pain, whether physical or psychological, and we anguish over our failings. Let us follow you now in recalling your passion and death. Teach us to follow you in our own passion and dying.*

Let us hear Jesus say, "Father, forgive them; they do not know what they are doing," and "Father, into your hands I commit my spirit." These could be the text on a poster for caregivers. Caregiving means dying just a little to ourselves so that our loved one may live just a little better life. We must forgive our loved ones when they "do not know what they are doing," and we must commit our own spirits into the hands of the Father if we are to do the work to which we are called.

Reflecting on the Way of the Cross for Caregivers:

- We caregivers are Simon of Cyrene, Veronica, Mary Magdalene and the other women, and the Beloved Disciple—faithful to the end and strengthened by Mary, Mother of Jesus and of us all.

- We are also Peter and the others, afraid and running away.
- And we are even Judas, sometimes betraying our loved one for our "right" to our own life.

Let me share with thee his pain
Who for all my sins was slain,
Who for me in torment died.
—Stabat Mater

Chapter 13

Giving Thanks

Jesus said, "Peace be with you," time after time when he appeared to the disciples after the Resurrection. How comforting Jesus' greeting must have been to Peter as he recalled his denial and to the apostles who had fled from Jesus when he was suffering and dying. Did not that same Jesus say to me as well, "Peace be with you," after Mother's death?

I am grateful for the privilege of caring for Mother during her final years.

Each year's Holy Week brings back her last days as I ponder Jesus' last days. One Holy Thursday, I imagined I was with Jesus and the disciples as Jesus washed their feet, and I questioned whether or not I had washed Mother's feet properly. When I insisted on continuing my own life by first working at Catholic Charities and then doing retreat work and always attending my religious community's meetings, was I merely being selfish or was I keeping myself sane so that I could serve Mother to the end? I could not know, nor will I ever know, whether my reasoning was correct. I do know that I was, through the entire time of caring for her, as psychologically healthy as I was at any time during my life.

As I write this little book, I am struck with the power of the caregiving experience. I wonder: What are the implications of this powerful experience for me who (I must admit) am now old and growing older? What does this all-consuming experience mean for all of us who care for others, even if we are not yet elderly or in need of care ourselves?

Having reflected on caring for Mother, with many wonderings, uncertainties and misgivings, I pray to my God in the spirit of Job (see Job 42:2-6):

> I know that you are all-powerful:
> What you conceive, you can perform.
> I am the one who obscured your designs
>   with my empty-headed words.
> I have been holding forth on matters I cannot understand,
>   on marvels beyond me and my knowledge.
> I knew you then only by hearsay;
>   but now, having seen you with my own eyes,
> I retract all I have said,
>   and in dust and ashes I repent.

Station XIII: Jesus is taken down from the cross

We adore you, O Christ, and we bless you;
Because by your holy cross, you have redeemed the world.

> *Dear Jesus, as we strive to follow your Way, we too have come to a time when we are confronted with intense suffering. We find it difficult to endure this pain, whether physical or psychological, and we anguish over our failings. Let us follow you now in recalling your passion and death. Teach us to follow you in our own passion and dying.*

Jesus is taken down from the cross. We will someday be relieved of our caregiving responsibilities. Neither of these are happy occasions, yet they do provide a curious relief: The pain of watching a loved one suffer is finally over. Yet we are left with an emptiness, a sorrow, a sense of guilt that we just cannot shake. How can this be the end? Is there no resurrection?

Reflecting on the Way of the Cross for Caregivers:

- How do we bridge from intense caregiving to "normal" life, when the death of the recipient of our care ends our ministry and when we, perhaps, are grieving ourselves?
- When the one we cared for dies, whatever we did or did not do recedes to the past.
- While we need to grieve and to work through regrets and even guilt, we need also to reach a place where we can ask forgiveness and forgive both the person we helped and ourselves before our God.
- Eventually, we need to treasure the privilege that was ours to accompany our loved one during his or her final journey to God.

Let me mingle tears with thee,
Mourning him who mourned for me,
All the days that I may live.

—Stabat Mater

Chapter 14

Picking Up the Pieces

My whole situation—my work at Catholic Charities and later in retreat ministry with older adults and my being with Mother—was one ministry. All of it resulted from prayerful discerning what God wanted of me at that particular time in my life. My time in prayer made this complex ministry possible—not easy, but possible. Moreover, I wanted to be with Mother to ease her last years.

That I was older at the time was a freeing factor in my decision. By "job" standards I was retirement age—sixty-nine when I went to live with Mother and seventy-four-and-a-half when she died. Such considerations as the ministry to which I should devote my life, my "career" development, a right to my own life, and even helping to support my congregation became minor issues and yielded to a more free, more relaxed approach to life and ministry when I went to live with her.

Moreover, as I prayed and looked to my older years, I realized that I needed to lessen administrative aspects of ministry. I had less psychological energy to cope with stress accompanying management and budget issues. Eventually I would need to reduce work time and, in the future, to retire.

These considerations freed me to leave Oakland Catholic Charities and move to Mother's Los Angeles home. When three years later my position in Los Angeles Catholic Charities ended, my own aging freed me again to begin a retreat ministry with older adults. Retreat ministry meshed with my prayer life and ministry to Mother, and in itself it was energizing. I was energized by the understanding, support and encouragement I received from my superiors, the group of Sisters with whom I met regularly, my spiritual director, and especially my sister. Before Mother's stroke, being with her was also energizing, comfortable and pleasant. I treasure our time together to this day, and I'm grateful that I could be with her.

What was de-energizing? Rather, I'd ask what was difficult and hard for me about caregiving? Mother's periods of agitation or disorientation frightened me. The fact that these times often occurred at night interfered with my own much-needed rest. But I have the gift of being able to sleep at will, and so I did not suffer from ill health.

No, the most difficult and heart-breaking aspect of caregiving was the last three weeks of Mother's life. She literally fought and begged to come home from the hospital and then the rehab/convalescent hospital. My often indirect conversation with others—especially my sister, who was my main support—and my constant prayer led me to make the decision that I could no longer care directly for Mother and, therefore, could not bring her home at the end.

This decision was never clear or obvious; it was simply the best decision I could make—even though I knew Mother felt that I was letting her down at the time of her greatest need. Prayer (including accepting and forgiving myself for my weakness and fright) literally, but barely, sustained me. At the end, and always in the five and a half years I was with Mother, somewhere underneath I sensed a fundamental peace, a feeling that God was with me and that this caregiving ministry was God's way for me.

Station XIV: Jesus is placed in the sepulcher

We adore you, O Christ, and we bless you;
Because by your holy cross, you have redeemed the world.

> *Dear Jesus, as we strive to follow your Way, we too have come to a time when we are confronted with intense suffering. We find it difficult to endure this pain, whether*

physical or psychological, and we anguish over our failings. Let us follow you now in recalling your passion and death. Teach us to follow you in our own passion and dying.

"Laid to rest." "Let perpetual light shine upon them." "May the souls of the faithful departed rest in peace. Amen." How comforting these words are for us caregivers who are left behind when our loved one dies. Jesus has been there before all of them and will welcome them into the next life. Yet we are left behind to pick up the pieces of our lives, now with the major focus of our lives for so many years suddenly gone.

Reflecting on the Way of the Cross for Caregivers:

- How does the powerful, all-consuming experience of giving care to another over a long period of time affect us? How do we want it to affect us?
- How might our caregiving experience affect the decisions we make in responding to God's call at another time?
- After our caregiving has ended, what about renewing our relationship with others? Can we accept them as they are? Will they accept us in a different role?
- If we ever need care, our own pain or weakness may make it almost impossible to accept it.

By the cross with thee to stay;
There with thee to weep and pray,
All I ask of thee to give.
—Stabat Mater

Chapter 15

Needing Care Ourselves

A few years after Mother's death, I was not reading signs at road intersections correctly, if at all. When I walked, I walked gingerly, lest I lose my balance. My head was dropping lower and lower until it rested on my chest. I was a bent old woman who could not stand up straight. It was the beginning of December, time to renew my driver's license. The eye test would tell me if my vision was adequate for driving. I passed all tests for the license, and it was renewed for five years.

In January, I fell. I promised myself I'd be more careful, but I fell several more times—always inside the house—and I always rose slowly but unhurt. Then, when the handle on a bag of groceries broke while I was going up the two stone stairs to the entryway of the house, I lost balance and fell on the stairs. Shaken but unhurt, I entered the house, lugging the groceries. Sometimes in the evening when I was eating dinner, reading, and watching TV, I would get lost when I rose to go to the kitchen—yes, actually lost. Focusing on the placement of the television, I would quickly reorient myself.

Then there was the night when, disoriented, I stood in the middle of the living room and focusing on the TV did nothing for what seemed like forever. Eventually, I began to pray, "Lord, this is it. I asked for help to face my own aging and to accept and live fully whatever might accompany it. Be with me now. Help me." Slowly, calm returned. I looked around and found myself. Actually, the Lord found me.

At the end of January, anxious and puzzled because of these physical changes, I drove to Pasadena for my monthly conference with my spiritual director. As always, her listening and reflective support strengthened me. As I was driving home, however, I noticed that I had difficulty seeing the direction cars approaching me were going. I knew the way well and did not need to read road signs, so I focused on driving in the center of the lane between the two lines that bound it and followed carefully the car in front of me. When I arrived home safely, I sat in the car and declared, "This has to be the last time I drive."

Giving up driving opened my mind, if not my heart, to many life-changing decisions. I prayed. I argued with myself. I tried to discern God's way for me at that moment. First, those who needed to know the changes in me should hear a full and honest disclosure. Second, I should not continue to live alone and therefore should move from Mother and Dad's house. Third, I must see my doctor.

I realized I was entering the last stage of my life, and I wanted to discern how God was inviting me to live it. The very striving to take steps prayerfully with God calmed me and helped me to be more objective, even while I continued to be very anxious and afraid. Over and over again I said to myself, "I don't understand."

Gradually, however, I thought through what was happening to me, drawing on the knowledge I had gained from caring for Mother. Slowly I realized that I could learn to adjust. I could help my mind interpret the changed images my eyes were receiving because of the different angle of vision. Just as a toddler can learn, after many falls, to stand, balance and walk, so I could learn to balance myself even when the forward thrust of my twelve-pound head was conditioning me to dive to the ground. I learned and am still learning. I haven't fallen for a long time. With the help of single vision lenses, I can even read the computer screen. I am more comfortable with myself.

In the meantime, the question of where I should move dominated my life because of both my own feelings and the perceptions of my superior, companions, friends and family. The first decision (there were others) was that I move *immediately* to our motherhouse health facility, where an excellent therapist would provide frequent physical therapy sessions. I could not agree to this decision: *immediately* was impossible. After a time, however, I agreed to move to a retirement community in California and, when I am frail and need care, move to our motherhouse in Adrian, Michigan. The delay would provide time and opportunity for me to adjust.

The decision and taking the necessary steps were not easy. But here I am, in Santa Cruz living at Dominican Oaks, a retirement facility of 200-plus apartments. Older men and women live here, including fourteen of us Adrian Dominican Sisters. Oaks residents are very welcoming, and the surrounding Santa Cruz community is home to many of our active sisters. I have already met one of my former students from the small high school in which I taught for nine years.

In small ways I am slowly accepting future frailty. Every so often, though, I hear myself say, "You don't have to walk so slowly yet" or "You can sit straighter." Sometimes these small gains in understanding and accepting are even fun. Knowing that we are progressing in accepting some physical diminishments might prepare us for receiving care in the future and, in time, for our dying.

I stood back in wonder when the moving van left Mother and Dad's home in Los Angeles. I relished the drive from Los Angeles to Santa Cruz along the Pacific coast past Santa Barbara and the approach to Dominican Oaks on Monterey Bay. As I looked out on a veritable forest of maple, pine, oak and birch trees from my apartment, I knew I was at home. In John 14:1-3, I read, "Do not let your hearts be troubled. Believe in God, believe also in me. In my Father's house there are many dwelling places. If it were not so, would I have told you that I go to prepare a place for you? And if I go and prepare a place for you, I will come again and will take you to myself, so that where I am, there you may be also."

I needed to take steps to improve my health. After inquiring from the Sisters and other residents, I eventually saw a primary physician. Based on her own diagnoses and directives, she referred me to physicians who specialized in physical medicine and in neurosurgery. Before long I was in surgery and screws and rods were bonding with bone to force the cervical vertebrae to hold my head erect. I had left Los Angeles and many doctor visits there thinking that my chin would always rest on my breast. Now I can actually look at a person with whom I am conversing; I can see the sky, the trees, and the beautiful flower beds. God is here in the people who made this possible, and in me. Truly magical and even mystical!

My journey to retirement has taught me to live in the present while treasuring the past. Loitering in the back of my consciousness is the future, the time when I may need further care. I can see myself at our motherhouse then. I can see myself leaving Santa Cruz and flying to Adrian, Michigan, by way of Detroit. I imagine being with the sisters who were in the novitiate with me.

Station XV: Jesus rises from the dead

We adore you, O Christ, and we bless you;
Because by your holy cross, you have redeemed the world.

> *Dear Jesus, as we strive to follow your Way, we too have come to a time when we are confronted with intense suffering. We find it difficult to endure this pain, whether physical or psychological, and we anguish over our failings. Let us follow you now in recalling your passion and death. Teach us to follow you in our own passion and dying.*

Now, let us caregivers join minds and hearts, if not hands, across the miles and walk to the foot of the Cross. Let us know the beauty that is there amid the ugly pain and disfigurement. Let us soak ourselves in the beauty that is love, dying for the ones we care for and for us. Let us trust and believe that this beauty will blossom and flame into the white heat and glory of the Resurrection. Alleluia!

Reflecting on the Way of the Cross for Caregivers:

- Whether we are old or young, our caregiving experience has a profound effect on us and can be a stimulus for growth in us.
- Be patient with the effects of the caregiving experience and open yourself to the influence and guidance of the Spirit.

- We too need to be cared for. We must accept that care.
- We will all rise from the dead, just as Jesus did.

Virgin of all virgins best!
Listen to my fond request;
Let me share thy grief divine.
—Stabat Mater

Stabat Mater Dolorosa

At the cross her station keeping,
Stood the mournful mother weeping,
Close to Jesus to the last.

Through her heart his sorrow sharing,
All his bitter anguish bearing,
Now at length the sword has passed.

O how sad and sore distressed,
Was that Mother highly blessed
Of the sole begotten Son.

Christ above in torment hangs,
She beneath beholds the pangs
Of her dying glorious Son.

Is there one who would not weep,
Whelmed in miseries so deep,
Christ's dear mother to behold?

Can the human heart refrain
From partaking in her pain
In that mother's pain untold?

Bruised, derided, cursed, defiled,
She beheld her tender child,
All with bloody scourges rent.

For the sins of his own nation
Saw him hang in desolation
Til his spirit forth he sent.

O thou Mother! Font of love,
Touch my spirit from above,
Make my heart with thine accord.

Make me feel as thou hast felt;
Make my soul to glow and melt
With the love of Christ my Lord.

Holy Mother pierce me through,
In my heart each wound renew
Of my Savior crucified.

Let me share with thee his pain
Who for all my sins was slain,
Who for me in torment died.

Let me mingle tears with thee,
Mourning him who mourned for me,
All the days that I may live.

By the cross with thee to stay;
There with thee to weep and pray,
All I ask of thee to give.

Virgin of all virgins best!
Listen to my fond request:
Let me share thy grief divine.

—attributed to Jacapone da Todi

Acknowledgments

I am grateful to those who have supported and encouraged me as I developed this book. In particular, I thank my brother, Justus George Lawler, who has offered invaluable suggestions. Members of my congregation, especially those with whom I have lived, my retreat partners, and many friends have listened patiently and expressed interest in the project. The residents of Dominican Oaks, where I now live, have enlarged and deepened my understanding of caregiving as I observe their gentle care for aging spouses and the kind help they extend to neighbors.

Gregory F. Augustine Pierce of ACTA Publications accepted this work for publication and edited it. I am especially grateful for his patience with me as I raised questions and made suggestions.

Bibliography for and about Caregivers

Attig, T. (2000) *The heart of grief; Death and the search for lasting love.* New York: Oxford University Press.

Bockelman, W. (1990) *Finding the right words; Offering care & comfort when you don't know what to say.* Minneapolis: Augsburg.

Boulden, J. & Boulden, J. (1991) *The caregiver's handbook.* Weaverville: Boulden.

Boulden, J. (1999) *A guide for caregivers; When death threatens.* Weaverville, CA: Boulden.

Byock, I. (1997) *Dying well; The prospect for growth at the end of life.* New York: Riverhead.

Davies, P. (1996) *When someone dies; What you can do.* San Luis Obispo: Sunnybank.

Dexter, P. (1999) *Coping as caregivers when a loved one is ill.* Mystic, CT: Twenty-Third.

Doka, K. (Ed.) (1997) *Living with grief; When illness is prolonged.* Washington: Hospice Foundation of America.

Eddy, R. & Eddy, K. (1997) *Writing with light; Meditations for caregivers in word and image.* Cleveland: United Church Press.

Editors at Fairview Press (1998) *Holiday hope; Remembering loved ones during special times of the year.* Minneapolis: Fairview Press.

Ferris, M. (1993) *Compassioning; Basic counseling skills for Christian care-givers.* Kansas City: Sheed & Ward.

Fitzgerald, H. (1994) *The mourning handbook.* New York: Simon & Schuster.

Franklin, A. & Sims, D. *Footsteps through grief.* Louisville: Grief Inc.

Gambill, A. (1994) *Do's and don'ts; Suggestions for the bereaved and their caregivers.* Colorado Springs: Bereavement.

Gilbert, R. (1999) *Finding your way after your parent dies; Hope for adults.* Notre Dame: Ave Maria Press.

Gilbert, R. (Ed.) (2002) *Healthcare & spirituality; Listening, assessing, caring.* Amityville: Baywood.

Golden, T. (1996) *Swallowed by a snake; The gift of the masculine side of healing.* Kensington, MD: Golden Healing.

Goldman, C. (2002) *The gifts of caregiving; Stories of hardship, hope, and healing.* Minneapolis: Fairview Press.

Grollman, E. & Grollman, S. (1997) *Your aging parents; Reflections for caregivers.* Boston: Beacon.

Grollman, E. & Kosik, K. (1996) *When someone you love has Alzheimer's; The caregiver's journey.* Boston: Beacon.

Grollman, E. (1995) *Caring and coping when your loved one is seriously ill.* Boston: Beacon.

Guntzelman, J. (1995) *124 prayers for caregivers.* Winona: St. Mary's Press.

Hamma, R. (2004) *In times of caregiving; Prayers of renewal & restoration.* Notre Dame: Ave Maria Press.

Hauerwas, S., Stoneking, C., Meador, K. & Cloutier, D. (Eds.) (2003) *Growing old in Christ.* Grand Rapids: Eerdmans.

Heidish, M. (1997) *Who cares? Simple ways YOU can reach out.* Notre Dame: Ave Maria.

Hodges, H. (1998) *Circle of years; A caregiver's journal.* Harrisburg: Morehouse.

Hover, M. (1993) *Caring for yourself when caring for others.* Mystic, CT: Twenty-Third.

Hutchison, J. & Rupp, J. (1999) *May I walk you home? Courage and comfort for caregivers of the very ill.* Notre Dame: Ave Maria.

Isle, S. (1996) *Giving care, taking care; Support for the helpers.* Maple Plain: Wintergreen.

Jevne, E. & Williams, D. (1998) *When dreams don't work; Profession-*

al caregivers and burnout. Amityville: Baywood.

Kottler, J. (2000) *Doing good; Passion and commitment for helping others.* Philadelphia: Brunner-Routledge.

Koven, M. & Pearl, L. (2004) *Mourning has broken; A collection of creative writing about grief and healing.* Toronto: KOPE.

Kuebelbeck, J. & O'Connor, V. (1995) *Caregiver therapy.* St. Meinrad: Abbey Press.

Luebering, C. (2002) *Dealing with the guilt after a difficult care decision.* St. Meinrad: Abbey Press.

Manning, D. (1984) *Comforting those who grieve; A guide for helping others.* San Francisco: Harper & Row.

Manning, D. (2001) *Thoughts for the holidays; Finding permission to grieve.* Oklahoma City: In-Sight.

Miller, J. & Cutshall, S. (2001) *The art of being a healing presence; A guide for those in caring relationships.* Fort Wayne: Willowgreen.

Miller, J. (1994) *How can I help? 12 things to do when someone you know suffers a loss.* Fort Wayne: Willowgreen.

Miller, J. (1995) *Autumn wisdom; Finding meaning in life's later years.* Minneapolis: Augsburg.

Miller, J. (1996) *The Caregiver's Book; Caring for another, caring for yourself.* Fort Wayne: Willowgreen.

Miller, J. (1997a) *One you love dying; 12 thoughts to guide you on the journey.* Fort Wayne: Willowgreen.

Miller, J. (1997b) *Welcoming change; Discovering hope in life's transitions.* Minneapolis: Augsburg

Miller, J. (1998) *The rewarding practice of journal writing; A guide for starting and keeping your personal journal.* Fort Wayne: Willowgreen.

Miller, J. (2002) *My Shepherd is the Lord; The timeless message of the 23rd Psalm.* Fort Wayne: Willowgreen.

Miller, J. (2003) *The art of listening in a healing way.* Fort Wayne: Willowgreen.

Morgan, R. (1994) *From grim to green pastures; Meditations for the sick and their caregivers.* Nashville: Upper Room.

Normile, P. (1995) *Prayers for care givers.* Cincinnati: St. Anthony Press.

Oliver, S. (1998) *What the dying teach us; Lessons on living.* Binghamton: Haworth.

Osmont, K. (2001) *What can I say and do?* Omaha: Centering.

Phillips, S. & Benner, P. (1994) *The crisis of care; Affirming and restoring caring practices in the helping professions.* Washington: Georgetown University Press.

Piva, S. (2004) *Hard questions for adult children and their aging parents; Facing the future together, with courage and compassion.* New York: Gotham.

Ramsey, N. (1998) *Pastoral diagnosis; A resource for ministries of care and counseling.* Minneapolis: Augsburg.

Ranieri, R. (2001) *Caring for yourself while caring for others.* Liguori, MO: Liguori.

Samples, P. (2001) *Comfort and be comforted; Reflections for caregivers.* Chicago: ACTA.

Sankar, A. (1999) *Dying at home; A family guide for caregiving.* Baltimore: Johns Hopkins University Press.

Sapienza, J. (2002) *Urgent whispers; Care of the dying (A personal reference manual for friends and family assisting a loved one at the end of life.* Eugene, OR: LLX Press.

Schreiber, E. (2001) *From one caregiver to another ... the hospice experience.* Westminster, PA: CP Martin.

Sims, D. (1993) *If I could just see hope.* Louisville: Grief Inc.

Smith, D. (1999) *Being a wounded healer; How to heal ourselves while we are healing others.* Madison: Psycho-spiritual publications.

Smith, H.I. (2002a) *Finding your way to say goodbye; Comfort for the dying and those who care for them.* Notre Dame: Ave Maria.

Smith, H.I. (2002b) *When you don't know what to say; How to help your grieving friends.* Kansas City: Beacon Hill Press.

Smith, H.I. (2004) *Grievers ask; Answers to questions about death and loss.* Minneapolis: Augsburg.

Sullivan, J. (2000) *The good listener.* Notre Dame: Ave Maria Press.

Thompson, G. (2002) *God knows caregiving can pull you apart; 12 ways to keep it all together.* Notre Dame: Sorin.

Van Bommel, H. (1996) *Caring for loved ones at home; An illustrat-*

ed guide to caring for loved ones who need short or long-term home care. Hantsport, Nova Scotia: Lancelot Press.
Van Bommel, H. (1993) *Choices; For people who have a terminal illness, their families and their caregivers.* Toronto: New Canada.
Weeks, O. D. & Johnson, C. (2000) *When all the friends have gone; A guide for aftercare providers.* Amityville: Baywood.
York, S. (2000) *Remembering well; Rituals for celebrating life and mourning death.* San Francisco: Jossey-Bass.
Zucker, R. (2002) *Family caregiving; When it wears you down.* St. Meinrad: Abbey Press.

This bibliography was prepared by The Reverend Richard B. Gilbert, Ph.D., BCC, CT, Director of Chaplaincy Services, Sherman Health Systems, Elgin, IL., and executive director, The World Pastoral Care Center. If you have questions or need additional assistance, you are welcome to contact him at dick.gilbert@shermanhospital.org.